MW00882813

THE ESSENTIAL HANDBOOK TO TURMERIC AND GINGER

THE ANTI-INFLAMMATORY DUO THAT WILL CHANGE YOUR LIFE

By

EVELYN CARMICHAEL

Evelyn Carmichael

INTRODUCTION

Many of us are more than happy to rely on prescribed medication to help us cure a wide variety of ills. But did you know that people all over the world have been using spices to help relieve and even cure a variety of conditions? Turmeric and ginger are two of the most powerful and commonly used spices that are known to fight inflammation, infections, and so much more.

Even though we in the western world are used to taking prescribed medications, some of us are just starting to discover the real benefits of these ancient yet highly nutritious spices.

Let this book show you the benefits of turmeric and ginger. Discover how you too can use the natural power of these spices to help you feel better and prevent a variety of ailments.

Let this book also show you how to use these ancient spices, and learn how to cook a few delicious meals and treats, that can help you benefit from the way they work.

Evelyn Carmichael

TABLE OF CONTENTS

Evelyn Carmichael

LEGAL NOTES

Disclaimer: All content of this handbook is created for educational and informational purposes. This author is not affiliated with any specific diet plan or weight loss strategy. Before any change of diet and exercise plan, it is recommended to consult your physician. Personal use of any content is to be taken at the sole risk of the individual. The author and publisher bare no responsibility therein.

Evelyn Carmichael

CHAPTER 1. THE HEALTH BENEFITS OF TURMERIC

Turmeric is thought to be one of the healthiest spices you'll come across. This spice, like ginger, contains a wide range of nutrients and compounds, and has incredible anti-inflammatory properties.

Turmeric's origin is from a plant found in southern Asia and India is still the world's largest source of the flavorful spice. In fact, it is the main spice used to make curry. But the root of the turmeric plant is the source of which medicine, food colorings, and even cosmetics can be originated from. With an active compound known as curcumin, this spice really has a lot going for it

Let's take a close look at just some of the health benefits of this wonderful spice:

Anti-inflammatory properties and absorption

Turmeric naturally contains over two dozen anti-inflammatory properties that can help to reduce swelling. Curcumin may well be the most powerful of the bunch, but is hard to get the amount you need and for your body to absorb it in the amounts found in curry recipes. To get the full benefits of the curcumin in Turmeric, it is recommended to use turmeric extract. Furthermore, recent studies have shown that to better absorb the turmeric extract, taking it with black pepper is extremely beneficial. While swallowing a couple of peppercorns may seem strange to you, be aware that some studies show absorption rates increasing to 2000%. Lately, you can find Turmeric (or labeled as curcumin) with black pepper together as an extract in the health food store.

Managing arthritis

Those who suffer from arthritis are frequently in pain, and turmeric can help. Thanks to the active properties found in curcumin, it can be used to help combat the associated pain and discomfort sufferers often feel. Incredibly, those who had taken curcumin as part of a trial were found to have a little less pain, and other symptoms.

Anticoagulant properties

Turmeric is thought to work as an anticoagulant by preventing platelets from sticking together, turmeric prevents blood clots from forming and remaining. This in turn, will help prevent heart attacks and strokes. Please speak to your doctor before you decide to use turmeric as an anticoagulant.

Antidepressant

Incredibly, it's thought that this lovely-tasting spice can work as an antidepressant. When used as part of a study in a laboratory, and on animals who were considered to be depressed, it was found that turmeric helped to relieve some of their symptoms. Furthermore, when this spice was used in human patients, it was thought that it has the same effect as Prozac when it comes to managing depression.

Lowering blood sugar levels

Adding a little bit of turmeric to your diet is thought to help reduce blood sugar levels in those with type 2 diabetes. It's also considered to be effective at helping to reverse some of the side effects that are associated with hyperglycemia, and insulin resistance. Those with type 2 diabetes should consider adding a little turmeric to their diet each day.

Alleviating pain

Turmeric extract is thought to have more anti-inflammatory agents that help relieve pain then many over the counter pain killers. In fact, many people use turmeric extract instead of an aspirin or other painkiller. While you should always take any pain medication that has been prescribed by your doctor, knowing that turmeric can help means you may be in a little less pain very soon.

Lowering cholesterol levels

We all know that the foods we consume can have a direct impact on our cholesterol levels. The good news is that turmeric can help to lower those levels. A study that took place, whereby individuals with high cholesterol were given turmeric showed that when they consumed turmeric daily, their cholesterol levels reduced slightly. In fact, several studies have shown that not only does turmeric extract reduce "bad" cholesterol, it also reduces the plaque build up in your arteries which is a significant cause of many heart issues and strokes.

Please note that if your doctor has prescribed you cholesterol-reducing medication, you should still take it.

Gastrointestinal issues

Anyone who suffers from gastrointestinal issues such as Crohn's disease, irritable bowel syndrome, or ulcerative colitis should consider consuming turmeric every day. The curcumin that's found in turmeric is thought to relieve the pain and discomfort experienced in these conditions, as well as acting as an anti-inflammatory. In some individuals who regularly consumed turmeric, it was found that they no longer needed to take the corticosteroids that were prescribed.

Please make sure you continue to take any mediation that your doctor prescribes you, even if you're feeling better.

Liver damage

Studies have shown that increasing your intake of curcumin each day could help to delay cirrhosis. This is all thanks to the anti-inflammatory and antioxidant effect that curcumin has. Those who currently suffer from liver damage should continue taking any mediation that has been prescribed to them by their doctor.

Alzheimer's Disease

Turmeric has also been shown to have positive uses in managing Alzheimer's Disease. Curcumin can speed up the clearance of amyloid protein plaques, reducing and the progression and symptoms of Alzheimer's.

Other uses:

Due to the amazing anti-inflammatory abilities you have read about that Turmeric/Curcumin contains, you will not be surprised that it has also been show to treat the following ailments:

- Fibromyalgia
- Rheumatoid Arthritis
- Skin conditions that cause pain or swelling such as ringworm
- Sprains or general swelling after injury
- Gum disease
- Inflammatory bowel disease
- Tuberculosis
- Urinary Bladder Infection
- Kidney Infection
- Prevention and treatment of cancers

-

CHAPTER 2. TURMERIC RECIPES

Let's take a look at some delicious turmeric recipes that will help you to get a little more of the spice in your diet every day.

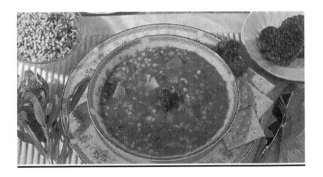

Moroccan style lentil soup

Serves: 12

Cooking time: 5 hours 30 minutes

Ingredients:

2 cups onions (Chopped)

2 tbsp lemon juice

2 cups carrots (Chopped)

½ cup cilantro (Chopped)

2 tsp extra virgin olive oil

4 cups spinach

1 tsp cumin

2 tbsp tomato paste

1 tsp coriander

1 can diced tomatoes

1 tsp turmeric

1 ¾ cups lentils

¼ tsp cinnamon

3 cups cauliflower (Chopped)

¼ tsp pepper

2 cups water

6 cups vegetable broth

Method:

Add the coriander, onions, pepper, turmeric, cumin, oil, garlic, and cinnamon to a slow cooker. Stir well, and add the lentils, broth, tomato paste, water, tomatoes, and cauliflower, and stir again. Place the lid on the slow cooker, and cook if for about 5 hours on a high heat, or 8 hours on a low heat, or until the lentils are soft.

30 minutes before the end of cooking, add the spinach, and stir well. A few minutes before the cooking time is up, add the lemon juice and cilantro, and stir. Serve.

Storage:

This soup should be kept in an airtight container in your refrigerator, and then heated gently in a pan before consuming.

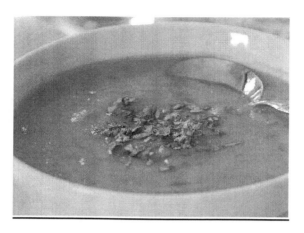

Mango Dal

Serves: 6

Cooking time: 40 minutes

Ingredients

1 cup lentils (Yellow)

½ cup cilantro (Chopped)

4 cups water

2 mangoes (Peeled, diced)

1 tsp salt

¼ tsp cayenne pepper

½ tsp turmeric

½ tsp coriander

1 tbsp canola oil

1 tbsp ginger (Minced)

½ tsp cumin seeds

4 cloves garlic (Minced)

1 onion (Chopped)

Method:

Rinse the lentils, and then add them to a pan along with the water, turmeric, and half the salt. Stir well, and bring to a boil. Now reduce the heat so the water starts to simmer, and cook for 15 minutes, covered, and stirring occasionally.

Now add the cumin seeds to a skillet along with some oil, and cook for about 30 seconds, or until they are starting to smell fragrant. Add the onion, and cook for 4-5 minutes, or until it starts to go soft. Add the coriander, pepper, ginger, garlic, and the rest of the salt, and stir well. Cook for 1 minute.

Add the garlic mix and the mangoes to the lentil mix, and stir well. Allow to simmer, and stir again. Cook for about 12-15 minutes, stirring occasionally, or until the lentils are breaking apart. Add some more cilantro, and serve.

Storage:

This Dal should be kept in an airtight container in your refrigerator, and then heated gently in a pan, or the microwave before consuming.

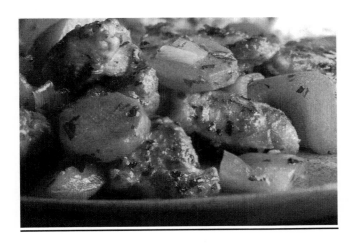

<u>Indian Style Chicken with Vegetables</u>

Serves: 4

Cooking time: 35 minutes

Ingredients:

2 tsp coriander

½ cup mint leaves (Chopped)

1 tsp cumin seeds

1 tbsp lime juice

1 tsp fennel seeds

3 red chilies (Dried)

1 tbsp corn starch

4 cloves of garlic (Sliced)

¾ tsp salt

1 red onion (Cubed)

½ tsp turmeric

1 green bell pepper (Cubed)

1 pound chicken breast (Boneless, skinless, cubed)

2 carrots (Chopped)

3 tbsp canola oil

Method:

Add the cumin, coriander and fennel to a pestle and mortar, and grind them until they resemble pepper. Now add them to a bowl, and place the turmeric, corn starch, and salt, and mix well. Add the chicken, and mix again, ensuring the meat gets covered in the spices.

Preheat a wok or skillet, on a high heat, and add 2 tbsp oil, along with the chicken and spices. Cook for about 5-8 minutes, or until the chicken is thoroughly cooked. Add the vegetables and stir, then add the mint and lime juice, stir again, and cook for about 30 seconds or until the vegetables are heated through. Serve.

Storage:

This dish should be kept in an airtight container in your refrigerator, and then heated gently in a pan or in the microwave before consuming. Please make sure the chicken is heated thoroughly before you consume it.

Evelyn Carmichael

CHAPTER 3. THE HEALTH BENEFITS OF GINGER

Ginger is thought to be one of the healthiest spices you can find. Containing a wide range of nutrients and compounds, this spice really is a super food.

When you scour the internet looking for healthy recipes, it's likely that many of them will contain ginger. This is because it's incredibly good for you, while also adding a nice flavor to a wide array of dishes too.

Let's take a close look at just some of the health benefits of this wonderful spice:

Anti-inflammatory properties

Ginger naturally contains a lot of anti-inflammatory properties that can help to reduce swelling. If you have some swelling, and you wish to get rid of it with or without the use of prescribed mediation, make sure you consume a little bit of ginger every day.

- Osteoarthritis

Those who suffer from osteoarthritis often feel a lot of stiffness and pain associated with this condition. In a trial consisting of more than 200 people with osteoarthritis, it was found that those who consumed ginger extract frequently were more likely to be in less pain than those who didn't.

Antioxidant properties

Ginger is a completely natural antioxidant, making it ideal if you would like to detox your body from harmful substances. It's also ideal if you simply want to stay healthy, and eat foods that can flush out toxins. The reason that ginger is so high in antioxidants is because it contains gingerol, which is a bioactive compound.

Great for morning sickness

If you or someone you know has morning sickness, you should be aware that ginger may help to combat it. Ginger has been shown to help to alleviate nausea, a common complaint with morning sickness. It's thought that 1.1 to 1.5 grams of ginger can help with these symptoms.

Great for sea sickness

If you're headed out to sea, and you know full well that you're going to suffer, take some ginger with you. Ginger has been used for many years by fishermen and sailors, who regularly spend a lot of time at sea. It's thought that 1.1 to 1.5 grams of ginger can help with the symptoms of sea sickness.

Lowering cholesterol levels

We all know that the foods we consume can have a direct impact on our cholesterol levels. The good news is that ginger can help to lower those levels. due to the anti-inflammatory properties that ginger possess, is thought to be good for your heart health overall. In specific to cholesterol, ginger activates an enzyme that increases your body's use of cholesterol and lowers it. A study that took place over a period of 6 weeks in individuals with high cholesterol showed that when they consumed just 3 grams of ginger powder a day, their "bad" cholesterol levels were lowered and their "good" cholesterol levels were higher.

Alleviating pain

While many people are more than happy to use painkillers to help them alleviate pain, there are others who are more than happy to take ginger as a painkiller. While you should always take any pain medication that has been prescribed by your doctor, knowing that ginger can help means you may be able to avoid over the counter painkillers for your ailments.

Ginger can help with muscle pain, and soreness too. It's thought that consuming about 2 grams of ginger every day for about 10-12 days can help to reduce chronic pain. Although the ginger you consume will not work right away, it is thought to have a cumulative effect of reducing inflammation, and therefore pain, after a few days, and more significantly within 10-12 days.

Helping to fight infections

In addition to containing anti-inflammatory and antioxidant properties, among others, ginger is also thought to be great at helping to fight infections. As we have already established it works as an antioxidant to flush out those nasty toxins, but this natural spice also works to inhibit bacteria growth.

If you suffer from gingivitis, consuming ginger each day is thought to help. But it's not just gingivitis sufferers who will benefit, those who have other infections could also find that ginger helps to ward them off too.

Reducing blood sugar levels

Although the research that has gone into the study of ginger and its ability to reduce sugar levels is fairly new, it is seen some significant results. Thought to be ideal at helping to reduce blood sugar levels in those with diabetes, consuming just 2 grams of ginger in powder form per day is considered very helpful. Recent research has shown that those with type 2 diabetes who consumed ginger everyday reduced their sugar level by twelve percent.

Although the study showed some promising results, those with diabetes should always take the medication they are prescribed.

31

Indigestion

If you occasionally suffer from indigestion, then ginger may be able to help you. Caused by the stomach delaying emptying itself, indigestion is thought to be relieved when ginger is consumed as the spice works to empty the stomach a little quicker. It's thought that just 1.2 grams of ginger in powder form consumed before a meal can help to speed up stomach digestion. If you have more frequent indigestion, be sure to see a doctor.

Menstruation pain

Some women suffer quite badly with menstruation pain, leading them to feel very uncomfortable each month. Did you know that ginger can help to bring a bit of pain relief? It's thought that consuming just 1 single gram of ginger powder can help due to the anti-inflammatory properties. The powder should be consumed for the first 3 days of the period, so it can get to work.

Working to prevent cancer

Ginger is thought to contain anti-cancer properties on a preventative and a therapeutic level. This includes properties in ginger that prevents and slows the progression of tumor growth.   This has prompted a lot of research on the claims that ginger can target specific cells to reduce inflammation and stimulate antioxidant pathways as well as free radicals and toxins in cancer cells.

Research has also been occurring on preventative measures of ginger on high risk individuals. A study of 30 people at high risk of colon cancer involved them consuming 2 grams of ginger extract each day. It was found that after the study, they had a lower chance of suffering from cancer.

Improving brain function

Some studies have shown that regular consumption of ginger can result in an improved brain function. It's also thought that consuming ginger can also help to prevent Alzheimer's disease.

Evelyn Carmichael

CHAPTER 4. GINGER RECIPES

Let's take a look at some delicious ginger recipes that will help you to get a little more ginger in your diet every day.

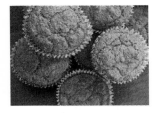

Carrot and Ginger Muffins

Serves: 12

Cooking time: 42 minutes

Ingredients:

Evelyn Carmichael

1 cup carrots (Grated)

2 tsp vanilla extract and

¼ tsp vanilla extract

1 egg

1 tbsp powdered sugar

½ cup coconut oil (Melted)

2 tbsp + 1 tsp vanilla almond milk (Unsweetened)

1/3 cup vanilla almond milk (Unsweetened)

½ cup apple sauce (Unsweetened)

¼ cup cream cheese (Softened)

¼ cup maple syrup

2 tbsp flax seeds

½ cup granulated sugar or sweetener

½ tsp baking soda

2 cups whole wheat flour

2 tsp baking powder

1 tsp cinnamon

½ tsp nutmeg

¾ tsp ginger (Ground)

Method:

Preheat your oven to 375 Fahrenheit. Spray 12 muffin cups with cooking spray or place a liner in each cup. Now add the carrots, apple sauce, honey, egg, coconut oil, 1/3 cup almond milk, and 2 tsp vanilla extract to a bowl. Stir well to combine. Add the sweetener, and whisk well.

Now add the cinnamon, salt, flour, nutmeg, ginger, baking soda, baking powder, and flax seeds to another bowl, and mix well. Pour these ingredients into the wet ingredients, and mix thoroughly. Now divide the mixture between the muffin cups, and cook for about 25 minutes, or until a tooth pick or small knife that's been inserted into the muffins comes out clean. Allow to cool.

Once the muffins are cooled, add the cream cheese, remaining almond milk, powdered sugar, and remaining vanilla extract to a bowl. Mix well. Once the mixture is nice and creamy, spread it over the top of the muffins and serve.

Storage:

Evelyn Carmichael

These should be kept in an airtight container, and enjoyed within 4-5 days. Alternatively, you may wish to store them in your freezer. Once frozen, the muffins can be gently defrosted over night or defrosted in the microwave.

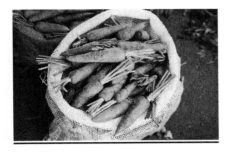

Roasted carrots with ginger and honey

Serves: 4-5

Cooking time: 45 minutes

Ingredients:

1 ½ pounds baby carrots (Peeled, with tops)

1 tbsp chives (Chopped)

1 tsp honey

Ground pepper

½ cup extra virgin olive oil

Sea salt

1 inch ginger, (Grated)

Method:

Preheat your oven to 425 Fahrenheit, and add the honey, oil, and ginger to a bowl. Stir well, and add the carrots, sprinkle the salt and pepper on top, and mix well. Cook the carrots in the oven for about 45-50 minutes, or until they are going a little brown at the edges. Serve.

Storage:

These carrots should be kept in an airtight container in your refrigerator, and then heated gently in a pan before consuming.

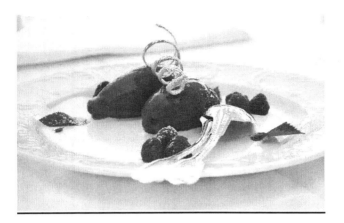

Blueberry and Ginger Sorbet with Lime

Serves: 4-5

Cooking time: 25 minutes

Ingredients:

5 cups blueberries (Washed)

2 tsp ginger (Grated)

¼ cup sugar or substitute

1 tsp lime zest

¼ cup honey

¼ cup lime juice

Method:

Add all of the ingredients to a blender, and blend until a liquid is formed, and the sorbet is a dark purple color. Place in your refrigerator for at least 2 hours, and then taste test the sorbet. Add more sugar if you need to. Now place the sorbet into an ice cream maker, and run the maker until the sorbet is thick and soft. This should take about 25 minutes.

Once the sorbet has the right consistency, place it in an airtight container, and store in your freezer until it's ready to be served.

Evelyn Carmichael

CHAPTER 5. COMBINING GINGER AND TURMERIC

Did you know that when you combine ginger and turmeric, you'll be combining two of the most powerful spices you can find? Used individually these spices will help to boost your health, and reduce pain and other conditions, but when you combine them, you can expect to gain even more benefits.

Working to prevent cancer

Ginger and turmeric are both thought to contain anti-cancer properties. Due to the high level of anti-inflammatories, ginger and turmeric have been researched for decades for their cancer fighting properties. In fact, the dynamic duo is thought to not only inhibit the growth of tumors but stop the cancer cells by causing cell "death" in cancer cells without

45

affecting healthy ones. Consuming both of these spices every day may well help to ward off cancer.

Tips

You have seen the advantages of taking Turmeric and ginger. Please be aware that while they are generally considered safe for consumption, like anything in your diet, don't overdo it. Follow the instructions from your health care professional and pay attention to the recommended doses on your extract bottle. Similarly, many extracts can cause complications and interactions with prescription medications. Make sure your doctor knows what supplements you are taking and the doses before you consume therapeutic levels of ginger and turmeric.

Start today!

Start by consuming more ginger and turmeric today, add a little more to your diet, and start to feel the benefits. I did, when I began consuming them for the very first time, just a few years ago. Now, I am less susceptible to a wide variety of conditions, and I generally just feel a little better too. If you don't care for the taste, check out your local health food store for supplements and powder forms. They are generally in a much more concentrated, therapeutic dose for specific ailments and will get you on your way to good health.

Evelyn Carmichael

CHAPTER 6. GINGER AND TURMERIC RECIPES

Let's take a look at some delicious ginger and turmeric recipes that will help you to get a little more in your diet every day.

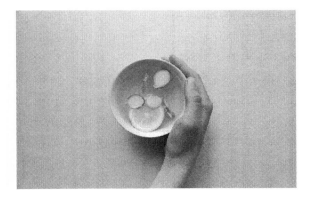

Turmeric and Ginger Tea

Serves: 1

Cooking time: 5 minutes

Ingredients:

1 tsp turmeric (Grated)

1 tsp ginger root

1 cup water

1 slice lemon

1 tsp honey

Method:

Add the water to a pan, and bring it to the boil. Now add the spices, and lower the heat. Simmer for 5 minutes, covered, and allow to cool. Add the honey and lemon once the tea is cool. Serve.

Storage:

This tea should be stored in the refrigerator and used within 3-4 days. Heat gently in a pan before drinking.

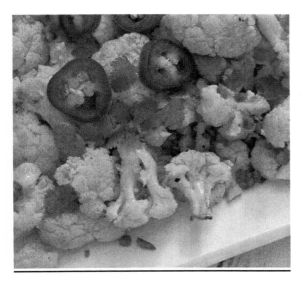

Cauliflower with Turmeric and Ginger

Serves: 4

Cooking time: 25 minutes

Ingredients:

3 tbsp vegetable oil

Salt

1 tbsp mustard seeds (Black)

1 cauliflower head (Chopped into florets)

1 jalapeno (Diced)

1 tsp turmeric

1 tbsp ginger (Grated)

Method:

Preheat your oven to 425 Fahrenheit. Now add the jalapeno, turmeric, ginger, mustard seeds, and oil to a bowl, and whisk well. Take the cauliflower, and add it to a baking dish, and toss with the mustard seed mix. Season, and add to the oven, and cook for about 25 minutes, or until the cauliflower is a little brown. Serve.

Storage:

This soup should be kept in an airtight container in your refrigerator, and then heated gently in a pan before consuming.

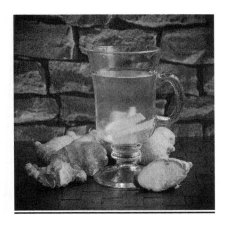

Turmeric and Honey delight

Serves: 1

Cooking time: 2 minutes

Ingredients:

½ cup honey

2 pinches black pepper (Ground)

2 tbsp ginger (Grated)

The zest of 1 lemon

2 tsp turmeric (Ground)

53

3-4 tbsp water

Method:

Add all of the ingredients to a bowl, and mix well.
Pour the mixture into a glass, and boil the water,
before pouring it into a jug. Allow it to cool a little, and
then add it to the glass. Stir well, and serve.

Storage:

This drink should be kept in an airtight container in
your refrigerator, and then heated gently in a pan
before consuming.

Read on for an excerpt of Evelyn Carmichael's book *The Essential Handbook to Apple Cider Vinegar*.

Evelyn Carmichael

THE ESSENTIAL HANDBOOK FOR APPLE CIDER VINEGAR

TIPS AND RECIPES FOR WEIGHT LOSS AND

IMPROVING YOUR HEALTH, BEAUTY, AND HOME

By

EVELYN CARMICHAEL

Copyright © 2016

Evelyn Carmichael

INTRODUCTION

Like me, you've walked into the supermarket a zillion times. How many times have you gone down the condiment aisle and seen apple cider vinegar and wondered, "So what's the difference?" At first glance, the only difference is the brown color and it is not as clear as the one you are used to picking up. Little do most people know that apple cider vinegar is jam-packed with some amazing uses.

Well, perhaps this is the right moment you should be reading this handbook. In it you will discover the essential uses and benefits of apple cider vinegar. Find out how you can use this all natural product for your home, in your beauty regime, for your health, and help you lose weight! All this and it is a common product you have probably had sitting on a shelf in your pantry for years! Discover how organic apple cider vinegar can lower blood sugar levels and aid other health issues such as high cholesterol, coughs and colds and poor digestion. It also provides a boost for your ever-fighting immune system.

Evelyn Carmichael

This Essential Handbook guides you uses of Apple Cider Vinegar in four main categories- to lose weight, your health, your body and beauty routine, and for your home. We will dive into these categories and you will learn tidbits like this amazing product provides an alternative to chemically produced cosmetics and therefore a gentle ingredient for your skin care routine. Also, each section has recipes on how to use for the particular remedy. As to your food, check out the recipe chapter. Apple cider vinegar gives your soups zest and lifts your sauces and salads plus some innovative recipes you will definitely want to try. Furthermore, apple cider vinegar is never outdone by household cleaners. Read on to see how Apple Cider Vinegar is your alternative to a more natural, environmentally-friendly and pet-friendly solution for your home and garden.

The Essential Handbook to Turmeric and Ginger

Evelyn Carmichael

EXCERPT
APPLE CIDER VINEGAR AND YOUR HEALTH

We are often reminded of the very old cliché "An apple a day, keeps the doctor away", an apt way to tell us of the importance of eating apples, or fruits, for that matter. This saying must have been coined because of the richness in nutrients found in apples. This is a wonder fruit as it acts on the body from two perspectives. One, the fruit is found to be moderately high in potassium which keeps your soft body tissues such as the muscles and arteries strong. This is why apples are such good anti-aging agent. On the other hand, apples are filled with calcium, that nutrient that maintains hard tissues such as your bones. For these reasons, ACV is considered high in the nutrients that come from the fruits that make it.

Help with Diabetes

While ACV is not a cure-all for illnesses, many people are able to attest to the benefits of the product in one way or another. In order to experience the true benefit, probably you should test it yourself. For example, ACV has been tested scientifically and found to reduce blood sugar levels. This is especially true in persons who have type 2 diabetes. Diabetes is a disease that occurs either because the body is resistant to the insulin it produces to control sugar in the blood, or it cannot produce the insulin to take care of the problem. Of course, if you have diabetes you well know you would be at great risk if you do not put a lid on the type of foods you eat, especially sugars. Apple Cider Vinegar has been shown to help reduce your blood sugar level, even when you haven't eaten exactly as you should. It has been found that just taking some ACV mixed with water improves the uptake of insulin in the body by between 19 – 34% especially when you have a meal high in carbohydrates. You would be surprised to know that two tablespoons of ACV taken before bedtime will cause your blood sugar to go down in the morning.

Help with High Cholesterol

High cholesterol levels in the body have been known to contribute heavily to heart disease and stroke. Furthermore, these diseases have been linked to high death rates. Although studies are limited, there is some scientific evidence that if you regularly ingest some ACV you would have a reduction in bad cholesterol. It is believed that the action of the antioxidant chlorogenic acid in ACV has much to do with preventing cholesterol deposits from crystalizing on the walls of your blood vessels, effectively lessening the deadly effects that can occur. A study that was done at Harvard University found that women who ate salads mixed with ACV had a reduced risk of heart disease than others who did not [2].

Help with Colds and Sinuses

What would many people give for a product that can relieve their sinus and cold symptoms? Many have been afflicted with sinus infections, sometimes seasonally, and there are those who will tell you it accompanies them throughout the year. Many will swear however that ACV does what regular medicine had not done for them. Some have gone to the point of ending their prescription medication. The potassium in ACV works to thin the mucus in the nasal passage while the acetic acid kills the germs that cause the problem to recur. Apple cider vinegar also has been used locally to ease and prevent the symptoms of the regular cold which causes such great misery on an average person of twice per year. A tablespoon of ACV will quickly dissolve the mucus and cause the nasal fluid to dry up. The solution also often takes care of a sore throat with just a gargle.

Help with Digestive Health Issues

Many people suffer from digestive problems, not to mention the very common acid reflux. This happens when the contents of the stomach flow back into the esophagus or food pipe. This can cause a real burning sensation and you get what is often called heart burn. Some persons also get this awful pain when they eat certain types of food. Apple cider vinegar has been found to provide tremendous relief from these digestive issues, especially when it is taken before a meal. A tablespoonful may be all you need to start eating your favorite foods that you had been avoiding.

Supports the Immune System

The immune system protects all other systems of the body against the invasion of harmful agents such as bacteria and viruses. The immune system itself however needs to be strengthened to carry out its work. Apple cider vinegar has long been used to provide this sort of boost to the immune system. There is the story that is often told of the thieves who survived the bubonic plague of the 1300s - 1700s in England because they drank a fermented vinegar brew made from herbs like rosemary, lavender and thyme. People in the villages and towns of England during the time of the bubonic plague also made stone crosses which they set up in the market places. The stone crosses were made with a depression which they filled with vinegar to drop coins in to kill the bacteria that caused the disease. This helped to stem the spread of the disease [3].

To own your copy of The Essential Handbook to Apple Cider Vinegar, please visit https://www.amazon.com/dp/B01NGYWEZE.

Evelyn Carmichael

ABOUT THE AUTHOR

Evelyn Carmichael

Evelyn was in the world of corporate finance before switching her life path after a successful battle with breast cancer. She is a personal life coach, fitness guru, and healthy lifestyle advocate.

Find out more on Facebook or at https://www.amazon.com/Evelyn-Carmichael/e/B01MQYHZLC

Evelyn Carmichael

OTHER BOOKS BY EVELYN CARMICHAEL

Evelyn is the author of the Essential Handbook Series.

Her titles include the following:

The Essential Handbook to Gluten Free Instant Pot Cooking

The Essential Handbook to Hashimoto's

The Essential Handbook to Hygge

The Essential Handbook to Superfood Smoothies

The Essential Handbook to Avocados The Superfood that Reduce Inflammation and lowers blood sugar, blood pressure, and your cholesterol

The Essential Handbook to Reversing Prediabetes and Diabetes: Meal Plans and Recipes to Reduce Your Blood Sugar Levels and Eliminate Diabetes and Prediabetes

The Essential Handbook to Turmeric and Ginger: The Anti-Inflammatory Duo that will Change your Life

The Essential Handbook to Coconut Oil: Tips, Recipes, and How to use for weight loss and in your daily life

<u>The Essential Handbook to Apple Cider Vinegar: Tips and Recipes for Weight Loss and Improving your Health, Beauty, & Home</u>

<u>The Art of Keeping Goals</u>

<u>The Essential Handbook for Choosing the Right Diet: A Guide to the Most Popular Diets and if They are Right for You</u>

<u>The Essential Handbook to Natural Living</u>

<u>The Essential Handbook to Essential Oils: Tips and Recipes for Weight Loss, Stress Relief, and Pain Management</u>

Knee Supports: Uses, Exercises, and Benefits

Evelyn Carmichael

AUTHOR NOTE

If you enjoyed this book, found it useful or otherwise then I'd really appreciate it if you would post a short review on Amazon. I do read all the reviews personally so that I can continually write what people are wanting.

Thanks for your support!

Evelyn Carmichael

Made in the USA
Middletown, DE
02 January 2018